DIABETIC DESTRUCTION

The medically proven framework for preventing and timing diabetes naturally

Jessie E. Jacque

Table of contents

Part one: Epidemic

Chapter one

What is an Epidemic

Plague alludes to an increment, frequently unexpected, in the quantity of instances of a sickness above what is typically anticipated in that populace around there. Episode conveys a similar meaning of scourge, however is frequently utilized for a more restricted geographic region. Bunch alludes to a collection of cases assembled, set up and time that are thought to be more prominent than the number expected, despite the fact that the normal number may not be known.

Pandemics happen when a specialist and vulnerable hosts are available in satisfactory numbers, and the specialist can be really passed from a source on to the helpless hosts. All the more explicitly, a scourge might result from:

- A new expansion in sum or destructiveness of the specialist.
- The new presentation of the specialist into a setting where it has not been previously.
- An improved method of transmission so more helpless people are uncovered.
- An adjustment of the weakness of the host reaction to the specialist, or potentially
- Factors that increment have openness or include presentation through new gateways of passage.

Scourges of irresistible sicknesses are for the most part brought about by a few variables remembering a tremendous change for the nature of the areal populace (e.g., expanded pressure perhaps extra explanation or expansion in the thickness of a vector animal types), the acquaintance of an arising microbe with an areal populace (by development of microorganism or host) or an unforeseen hereditary change that is in the microorganism repository.
For the most part, scourges worry with the examples of irresistible illness spread.An pestilence might happen when resistance to either a laid out microbe or recently arising novel microorganism is abruptly diminished underneath that found in the endemic harmony and the transmission limit is surpassed.

For instance, in meningococcal diseases, an assault rate of more than 15 cases for every 100,000 individuals for two continuous weeks is viewed as a scourge.

A pestilence might be limited to one area inside one nation or further foster more areas in a nation, in any case, on the off chance that it spreads to other local nations or even among landmasses however provided that effects or compromises a significant number of populace, it could be supervised as inside the particulars of pandemic. The enlisting and reporting of plague for the most part requires a decent comprehension of a pattern pace of rate; scourges for specific illnesses, like flu, are characterized as arriving at some characterized expansion in frequency over this baseline.A few instances of an exceptionally uncommon illness might be delegated a pandemic, while many instances of a typical illness (like the normal cold) wouldn't. A pestilence can cause gigantic harm through monetary and financial misfortunes notwithstanding hindered wellbeing and death toll.

Chapter two:

How type 2 Diabetes turned into an Epidemic

This idea has been remembered to incline toward anastomotic break and wound disturbance. The expansion in the degrees of proinflammatory cytokines brings about a deficient resistant reaction to microorganisms and vascular aggravation, in this way adding to less fortunate careful results

Diabetes is viewed as a 21st-century scourge that influences numerous persistent sicknesses. In any case, studies connecting diabetes to more unfortunate careful results, particularly in esophageal medical procedures, are restricted. Diabetes can prompt different serious complexities, for example, coronary course illness, lower furthest point arteriopathy, retinopathy and diabetic nephropathy, which influence the existence of a huge populace around the world. The quick development of diabetes represents a disturbing weight on worldwide social and financial turn of events.

In the last many years, type 2 diabetes (T2D) has turned into an enormous and consistently developing danger and one of the main general medical problems in essentially every locale of the world.

As per the National Health InterviewSurvey (NHIS), the predominance of analyzed diabetes multiplied from 1990 to 2016 (3.5% to 9.7%). In China, the pervasiveness of diabetes additionally expanded quickly from under 1% in 1980 to 11.2% in 2018. The danger was reliably misjudged on the grounds that a significant extent stayed undiscovered.

The expectation from the International Diabetes Federation is that 600 million individuals overall will be living with diabetes in 2035. A high rate of diabetes-specific entanglements, like kidney disappointment and fringe vein illness, seriously affects personal satisfaction in diabetic patients.

In 1994, the head of the Centers for Disease Control and Prevention's (CDC) diabetes program proclaimed that diabetes had arrived at a pandemic extent and ought to be considered as a significant general medical condition.

While diabetes mortality is ascending for all race and pay gatherings, confusions and higher demise rates happen especially among minorities and low-pay gatherings, in this way worsening wellbeing variations. Diabetes is a pandemic. The high and quickly expanding commonness of the sickness requests this portrayal.

Chapter three

The distinction between Type 1 and type 2 Diabetes

Type 2 diabetes isn't equivalent to Type 1 diabetes. In Type 1 diabetes, your pancreas makes no insulin. In Type 2, your pancreas doesn't make sufficient insulin, and the insulin it is making doesn't necessarily function as it ought to. The two kinds are types of diabetes mellitus, meaning they lead to hyperglycemia (high glucose).

Type 2 diabetes generally influences more established grown-ups, however it's turning out to be more normal in kids. Type 1 diabetes normally creates in kids or youthful grown-ups, yet individuals of all ages can get it.

Who is in danger of creating Type 2 diabetes?

You're bound to foster Type 2 diabetes on the off chance that you:

- Are Black, Hispanic, American Indian, Asian American or Pacific Islander.
- Are more established than 45.
- Are overweight/weight.
- Try not to work out.
- Had gestational diabetes while pregnant.
- Have a family background of diabetes.
- Have hypertension.
- Have prediabetes (higher than typical glucose, however not sufficiently high to be Type 2 diabetes).

How normal is Type 2 diabetes?
Type 2 diabetes is the most widely recognized type of diabetes. Around 1 of every 10 Americans have the infection. It's the seventh driving reason for death in the U.S.

EFFECTS AND CAUSES

What causes Type 2 diabetes?

Type 2 diabetes is created when the pancreas makes less insulin than the body needs, and the body cells quit answering insulin. They don't accept sugar as they ought to. Sugar develops in your blood. At the point when cells don't answer insulin, this is called insulin obstruction. It's generally brought about by:
Way of life factors, including heftiness and an absence of activity.
Hereditary qualities, or strange qualities, that keep cells from filling in as they ought to.

What are the side effects of Type 2 diabetes?
Side effects of Type 2 diabetes will generally foster gradually after some time. They can include:

- Obscured vision.
- Weariness.
- Feeling exceptionally eager or parched.
- Expanded need to pee (as a rule around evening time).
- Slow recuperating of cuts or injuries.
- Shivering or deadness in your grasp or feet.
- Unexplained weight reduction.

What are the complexities of high glucose levels?

Possible complexities of high glucose levels from Type 2 diabetes can include:

- Stomach related issues, including gastroparesis.
- Eye issues, including diabetes-related retinopathy.
- Foot issues, including leg and foot ulcers.
- Gum sickness and other mouth issues.
- Hearing misfortune.
- Coronary illness.
- Kidney sickness.
- Liver issues, including nonalcoholic greasy liver sickness.
- Fringe neuropathy (nerve harm).
- Sexual brokenness.
- Skin conditions.Stroke.
- Urinary parcel contaminations and bladder diseases.

Once in a while, Type 2 diabetes prompts a condition called diabetes-related ketoacidosis (DKA). DKA is a dangerous condition that makes your blood become acidic. Individuals with Type 1 diabetes are bound to have DKA.

Determination AND TESTS

How is Type 2 diabetes analyzed?

- The accompanying blood tests assist your medical services supplier with diagnosing diabetes:

- Fasting plasma glucose test: checks your blood glucose level. This test is best finished in the workplace in the first part of the day following an eight hour quick (nothing to eat or drink aside from tastes of water).

- Irregular plasma glucose test: This lab test should be possible any time without the need to be quick.

- Glycosylated hemoglobin testing (A1c) measures your typical glucose levels for more than 90 days.

- Oral glucose resilience testing checks your glucose levels when you drink a sweet refreshment. The test assesses how your body handles glucose.

Kind of test

- Fasting glucose test Diabetes (mg/dL) 126 or higher Random (whenever).
- Glucose test Diabetes (mg/dL) 200 or higher.
- A1c test Diabetes (mg/dL) 6.5% or higher.
- Oral glucose resilience test Diabetes (mg/dL) 200 or higher.

The executives AND TREATMENT

How is Type 2 diabetes made due?

There's no remedy for Type 2 diabetes. However, you can deal with the condition by keeping a solid way of life and taking prescriptions if necessary. Work with your medical care supplier to deal with your:

- Glucose: A blood glucose meter or consistent glucose checking (CGM) can assist you with meeting your glucose target. Your medical services supplier may likewise suggest normal A1c tests, oral drugs (pills), insulin treatment or injectable non-insulin diabetes prescriptions.

- Pulse: Lower your circulatory strain by not smoking, practicing consistently and eating a solid eating regimen. Your medical care supplier might suggest pulse prescriptions like beta blockers or ACE inhibitors.

- Cholesterol: Follow a dinner plan low in immersed fats, trans fat, salt and sugar. Your medical services supplier might suggest statins, which are a sort of medication to bring down cholesterol.

What should a Type 2 diabetes feast plan incorporate?

Ask your medical services supplier or a nutritionist to suggest a dinner plan that is ideal for you. As a rule, a Type 2 diabetes dinner plans ought to include:

- Lean proteins: Proteins low in immersed fats incorporate chicken, eggs and fish. Plant-based proteins incorporate tofu, nuts and beans.

- Negligibly handled carbs: Refined carbs like white bread, pasta and potatoes can cause your glucose to rapidly increment. Pick carbs that cause a more slow glucose increment, for example, entire grains like cereal, earthy colored rice and entire grain pasta.

- No additional salt: Too much sodium, or salt, can expand your pulse. Bring down your sodium by keeping away from handled food varieties like those that come in jars or bundles. Pick sans salt flavors and utilize sound oils rather than salad dressing.

- No additional sugars: Avoid sweet food sources and beverages, like pies, cakes and pop. Pick water or unsweetened tea to drink.

- Non-boring vegetables: These vegetables are lower in carbs, so they don't cause glucose spikes. Models incorporate broccoli, carrots and cauliflower.

Will I really want medicine or insulin for Type 2 diabetes?

Certain individuals take drugs to oversee diabetes, alongside diet and exercise. Your medical services supplier might suggest oral diabetes prescriptions. These are pills or fluids that you take by mouth. For instance, a medication called metformin helps control how much glucose your liver produces.

You can likewise take insulin to assist your body with utilizing sugar all the more productively. Insulin comes in the accompanying structures:

- Injectable insulin is a shot you give yourself. A great many people infuse insulin into a plump piece of their body like their gut. Injectable insulin is accessible in a vial or an insulin pen.

- Breathed in insulin is breathed in through your mouth. It is just accessible in a quick acting structure.

- Insulin siphons convey insulin persistently, like how a solid pancreas would. Siphons discharge insulin into your body through a little cannula (meager, adaptable cylinder). Siphons interface with a mechanized gadget that allows you to control the portion and recurrence of insulin.

Counteraction

How might I forestall Type 2 diabetes?
You can forestall or defer Type 2 diabetes by:

- Eating a sound eating regimen.
- Working out.
- Shedding pounds.
- Normal tests and screenings with your medical care supplier can likewise assist you with holding your glucose under control.

Viewpoint/PROGNOSIS

What is the viewpoint for Type 2 diabetes?

In the event that you have Type 2 diabetes, your viewpoint relies heavily on how well you deal with your blood glucose level. Untreated Type 2 diabetes can prompt a scope of perilous medical issues. Diabetes requires long lasting administration.

When would it be a good idea for me to call my PCP?

It's critical to screen diabetes intently assuming you're wiped out. Indeed, even a typical virus can be risky on the off chance that it obstructs your insulin and glucose levels. Make a "day off" plan with your medical services supplier so you know how frequently to check your glucose and what drugs to take.

Contact your supplier immediately on the off chance that you experience:

Disarray or cognitive decline.

Fever of 100°F or higher.

- High glucose for over 24 hours.
- Sickness and retching for over four hours.
- Issues with equilibrium or coordination.
- Extreme agony takes place in your body.
- Inconvenience moving your arms or legs.

PS Type 2 diabetes is an illness where your body doesn't make sufficient insulin and can't utilize sugar the manner in which it ought to. Sugar, or glucose, develops in your blood. High glucose can prompt serious unexpected problems. However, Type 2 diabetes is sensible. Normal activity and a solid eating regimen can assist you with dealing with your glucose. You may likewise require medicine or insulin. Assuming you have Type 2 diabetes, you ought to screen your glucose at home consistently and remain nearby with your medical care supplier.

The critical difference between type 1 and type 2 diabetes is that type 1 is accepted to be brought about by an immune system response and grows from the get-go throughout everyday life. Type 2 diabetes is created

throughout numerous years and is connected to way of life factors, for example, being idle and conveying overabundance weight. It's normally analyzed in grown-ups.

Risk factors for type 1 diabetes are not as clear, but rather family ancestry might assume a part.

Reasons for type 1 diabetes
The body's invulnerable framework is liable for warding off unfamiliar intruders, for example, destructive infections and bacteria.Type 1 diabetes is accepted to be brought about by an immune system response. In individuals with type 1 diabetes, the safe framework confuses the body's own solid cells with unfamiliar trespassers.

The safe framework assaults and obliterates the insulin-creating beta cells in the pancreas. After these beta cells are annihilated, the body can't create insulin.

Scientists don't have the foggiest idea why the invulnerable framework now and again goes after the body's own cells. It might have something to do with hereditary and natural variables, for example, openness to infections.
Investigation into immune system illnesses is progressing. Diet and way of life propensities don't cause type 1 diabetes.

Reasons for type 2 diabetes
Individuals with type 2 diabetes have insulin obstruction. The body actually creates insulin, however it cannot utilize it really.
Specialists don't know why certain individuals become insulin safe and others don't, however a few lifestyle elements might contribute, including being idle and conveying overabundance weight.
Other hereditary and ecological variables may likewise assume a part. At the point when you foster sort 2 diabetes, your pancreas will attempt to repay by delivering more insulin. Since your body can't really utilize insulin, glucose gathers in your circulatory system.

How does diabetes influence the body?

There are two fundamental sorts of diabetes: type 1 and type 2.

The two kinds of diabetes are constant illnesses that influence the manner in which your body manages glucose or glucose. Glucose is the fuel that takes care of your body's cells, yet to enter your cells it needs a key. Insulin is simply key.
Individuals with type 1 diabetes don't deliver insulin. You can consider it not having a key.
Individuals with type 2 diabetes don't answer insulin as well as they ought to and later in the illness frequently don't make sufficient insulin. You can consider it having a wrecked key.
The two kinds of diabetes can prompt persistently high glucose levels. That builds the gamble of diabetes confusions.

What are the gamble factors for type 1 and type 2 diabetes?
Risk factors for type 1 diabetes are less clear than risk factors for type 2 diabetes.
Realized risk factors include:

Family ancestry: People with a parent or kin with type 1 diabetes have a higher gamble of creating it themselves.

Age: Type 1 diabetes can show up at whatever stage in life, however it's generally normal among youngsters and youths.
Type 2 diabetes risk factors
You're in danger of creating type 2 diabetes in the event that you:
Have prediabetes, or marginally raised glucose levels are conveying overabundance weight or are corpulence.
Have a great deal of gut fat are genuinely dynamic under 3 times each week

- Are over age 45 Has at any point had gestational diabetes, which is diabetes during pregnancy.Have brought forth a child weighing in excess of 9 pounds.

- Are Black, Hispanic or Latino, American Indian, or Alaska Native because of underlying imbalances adding to wellbeing variations.

- Have a close relative with type 2 diabetes.
- Have polycystic ovary disorder (PCOS).

What are the side effects of diabetes?
On the off chance that not made due, type 1 and type 2 diabetes can prompt side effects, for example,

- Peeing every now and again.
- Feeling extremely parched and drinking a ton.
- Feeling extremely eager.
- Feeling extremely exhausted.
- Having foggy vision.
- Having cuts or injuries that don't mend as expected.
- Having exceptionally dry skin.
- Having more contaminants than expected.

Individuals with type 1 and type 2 diabetes may likewise encounter touchiness, state of mind changes, and unexpected weight loss.Diabetes and deadness in hands and feet
Individuals with type 1 and type 2 diabetes might encounter deadness and shivering in their grasp or feet. Great glucose the executives altogether diminishes the gamble of creating deadness and shivering in somebody with type 1 diabetes, as per the American Diabetes Association (ADA).

Albeit a large number of the side effects of type 1 and type 2 diabetes are comparative, they present in totally different ways.
Many individuals with type 2 diabetes will not have side effects for a long time, and their side effects frequently foster gradually over an extensive stretch of time.
Certain individuals with type 2 diabetes have no side effects by any means and don't find they have the condition until confusions emerge.

The side effects of type 1 diabetes grow rapidly, commonly throughout a little while.
When known as adolescent diabetes, this type normally creates in youth or immaturity. In any case, creating type 1 diabetes sometime down the road is conceivable.

How are type 1 and type 2 diabetes treated?
There's at present no remedy for type 1 diabetes. Individuals with type 1 diabetes don't deliver insulin, so it should be consistently taken, and glucose levels should be routinely checked.

Certain individuals bring infusions into delicate tissue, like the stomach, arm, or backside, a few times each day. Others use insulin siphons. Insulin siphons supply a consistent measure of insulin into the body through a little cylinder.

Glucose testing is a fundamental piece of overseeing type 1 diabetes since glucose levels can go all over rapidly.

Type 2 diabetes can be overseen and, surprisingly, forestalled with diet and exercise, yet many individuals need additional help. On the off chance that way of life changes aren't sufficient, your primary care physician might recommend prescriptions that assist your body with utilizing insulin all the more actually.
Observing your glucose is a fundamental piece of type 2 diabetes the executives, as well. It's the best way to realize whether you're meeting your objective levels.
Your PCP might suggest testing your glucose periodically or all the more oftentimes. On the off chance that your glucose levels are high, your primary care physician might suggest insulin infusions.

Might diabetes at any point be forestalled?
Type 1 diabetes can't be forestalled.

It could be feasible to bring down your gamble of creating type 2 diabetes through these way of life changes, for example,

- Keeping a moderate weight.
- Working with your primary care physician to foster a sound weight reduction plan, on the off chance that you are overweight.
- Expanding your action levels.
- Eating a decent eating regimen and diminishing your admission of sweet food sources or excessively handled food sources.

Regardless of whether you can't forestall the illness, cautious checking can get your glucose levels back to standard and forestall the improvement of serious inconveniences.

How normal is diabetes?

As per the Centers for Disease Control and Prevention (CDC), 37.3 million individuals in the United States have diabetes. That is somewhat more than 1 of every 11 individuals.

The CDC assesses that 8.5 million individuals are living with undiscovered diabetes. That is around 3.4 percent of all U.S. grown-ups.
The level of individuals with diabetes increments with age. Among those 65 years of age and more seasoned, the rate arrives at 29.2 percent.

Are men bound to get diabetes?
People get diabetes at generally a similar rate.

Yet, commonness rates are higher among specific races and identities in the United States.
Measurements show that diabetes happens all the more every now and again among generally underestimated populaces in the United States.
Research recommends that this might be expected to some extent to ecological elements, like the historical backdrop of unfair lodging and loaning approaches in the United States.
Specialists say that these strategies came about in racially and ethnically isolated areas that have deficient admittance to good food sources, lacking well being instructive assets, and higher paces of weight — a gamble factor for type 2 diabetes.

Native American and Alaska Native grown-ups are just multiple times more probable than non-Hispanic white grown-ups to be determined to have diabetes.
For all kinds of people, diabetes analysis is most noteworthy among American Indians and Alaska Natives, non-Hispanic blacks, and individuals of Hispanic origin.
Commonness rates are higher for Hispanic Americans of Mexican or Puerto Rican plunge than they are for those of Central and South American or Cuban plummet.
Among non-Hispanic Asian Americans, individuals with Asian Indian and Filipino lineage have higher rates of diabetes than individuals with Chinese or other Asian heritages.

How normal is type 1 diabetes

Type 1 diabetes is more uncommon than type 2.

Around 5 to 10 percent of individuals with diabetes have type 1. It typically occurs in kids, adolescents, and youthful grown-ups — however can occur at whatever stage in life.

How normal is type 2 diabetes?
Type 2 diabetes is considerably more typical than type 1, and 90 to 95 percent of individuals with diabetes have type 2.

Which diets are suggested for diabetes?
Healthful administration and dealing with your glucose are vital to living with diabetes.

On the off chance that you have type 1 diabetes, work with your primary care physician to distinguish how much insulin you might have to infuse in the wake of eating particular sorts of food.

For instance, certain starches can cause glucose levels to increment in individuals with type 1 diabetes rapidly. You'll have to neutralize this by taking insulin, yet you'll have to know how much insulin to take. Study type 1 diabetes and diet.

Individuals with type 2 diabetes need to zero in on smart dieting.

Weight reduction is much of the time a section of type 2 diabetes treatment plans. A specialist or nutritionist might suggest a low-calorie dinner plan. This could mean decreasing your utilization of creature fats and low quality food.
Normally, individuals with type 2 diabetes or prediabetes are prescribed to diminish their utilization of handled food varieties, trans fat, sweet beverages, and liquor.
Individuals with diabetes might have to attempt various eating regimens and dietary intends to track down that employer , their wellbeing, way of life, and financial plan.

The principal distinction between type 1 and type 2 diabetes is that type 1 diabetes is a hereditary condition that frequently appears right off the bat throughout everyday life, and type 2 is predominantly way of life related and creates after some time. With type 1

diabetes, your resistant framework is going after and annihilating the insulin-delivering cells in your pancreas.
In spite of the fact that type 1 and type 2 diabetes both share things practically speaking, there are bunches of contrasts. Like what causes them, who they influence, and how you ought to oversee them.

For a beginning, type 1 influences 8% of everybody with diabetes. While type 2 diabetes influences around 90%.

Certain individuals get confused between type 1 and type 2 diabetes. This can mean you need to make sense of the fact that what works for one kind doesn't work for the other, and that there are various causes.
The primary thing to recollect is that both are basically as serious as one another. Having high blood glucose (or sugar) levels can prompt serious unexpected problems, regardless of whether you have type 1 or type 2 diabetes. So on the off chance that you have either condition, you really want to find the correct ways to oversee it.

Chapter four

The entire Body Effect

Glucose is a frequently underrated part of your wellbeing. At the point when it's out of equilibrium over an extensive stretch of time, it could form into diabetes.

Diabetes influences your body's capacity to create or utilize insulin, a chemical that permits your body to turn glucose (sugar) into energy.

Here are what side effects might happen to your body when diabetes creates.
Diabetes can be successfully overseen when analyzed early. In any case, when left untreated, it can prompt potential confusions that include:

- Coronary illness
- Stroke
- Kidney harm
- Nerve harm

Regularly after you eat or drink, your body will separate sugars from your food and use them for energy in your cells.

To achieve this, your pancreas needs to create a chemical called insulin. Insulin works with the most common way of pulling sugar from the blood and placing it in the cells for use, or energy.
Assuming you have diabetes, your pancreas either creates too little insulin or none by any means. The insulin can't be utilized really.
This permits blood glucose levels to ascend while your other cells are denied much-required energy. This can prompt a wide assortment of issues influencing practically every significant body framework.

Kinds of diabetes
The impacts of diabetes on your body likewise relies upon the sort you have. There are two, fundamental kinds of diabetes: type 1 and type 2.

- Type 1, likewise called adolescent diabetes or insulin-subordinate diabetes, is a safe framework problem. Your own resistant framework goes after the insulin-delivering cells in the pancreas, obliterating your body's capacity to make insulin. With type 1 diabetes, you should accept insulin to live. A great many people accept their sort 1 finding as a kid or youthful grown-up.

- Type 2 is connected with insulin obstruction. It used to happen in more established populaces, yet presently more youthful populaces are creating type 2 diabetes. This is a consequence of specific way of life, dietary, and exercise propensities.

With type 2 diabetes, your pancreas quits utilizing insulin actually. This causes issues with having the option to maneuver sugar from the blood and put it into the cells for energy. Ultimately, this can prompt the requirement for insulin medicine.
You can successfully oversee prior stages like prediabetes with a reasonable eating regimen, work out, and cautious observing of blood sugars. This can likewise forestall the advancement of type 2 diabetes.

Diabetes can be controlled. Now and again, it might go into abatement if necessary way of life changes are made.
Gestational diabetes is high glucose that is created during pregnancy. More often than not, you can oversee gestational diabetes through diet and exercise. It likewise commonly settles after the child is conveyed.
Gestational diabetes can expand your gamble of intricacies during pregnancy. It can likewise build the gamble of type 2 diabetes improvement further down the road for both the birthing guardian and youngster.

Endocrine, excretory, and stomach related frameworks
In the event that your pancreas creates almost no insulin or on the other hand on the off chance that your body can't utilize it, different chemicals are utilized to transform fat into energy. This can make elevated degrees of poisonous synthetics, including

acids and ketone bodies, which might prompt a condition called diabetic ketoacidosis.
Diabetic ketoacidosis is a serious confusion of the illness. Side effects include:

- Outrageous thirst
- Unnecessary pee
- Weakness

Your breath might have a pleasant fragrance that is brought about by the raised degrees of ketones in the blood. High glucose levels and abundance of ketones in your pee can affirm diabetic ketoacidosis. On the off chance that untreated, this condition can prompt loss of cognizance or even passing.

Diabetic hyperglycemic hyperosmolar disorder (HHS) happens in type 2 diabetes. It includes extremely high blood glucose levels however no ketones.
You could become dried out with this condition. You might try and pass out. HHS is most normal in individuals whose diabetes is undiscovered, or who haven't had the option to deal with their diabetes well. It can likewise be brought about by a coronary failure, stroke, or contamination.
High blood glucose levels might cause gastroparesis. This is the point at which it's difficult for your stomach to purge totally. This deferral can cause blood glucose levels to rise. Subsequently, you may likewise insight:

- Sickness
- Regurgitating
- Bulging
- Indigestion
- Kidney harm

Diabetes can likewise harm your kidneys and influence their capacity to channel side-effects from your blood. On the off chance that your primary care physician identifies microalbuminuria, or raised measures of protein in your pee, it very well may be an indication that your kidneys aren't working as expected.

Kidney illness connected with diabetes is called diabetic nephropathy. This condition doesn't show side effects until its later stages.
On the off chance that you have diabetes, your PCP will assess you for nephropathy to assist with forestalling irreversible kidney harm or kidney disappointment.

Circulatory framework
Diabetes raises your gamble of growing hypertension, which overburdens your heart.
At the point when you have high blood glucose levels, this can add to the arrangement of greasy stores in vein walls. After some time, it can confine blood stream and increase the gamble of atherosclerosis, or solidifying of the vein. As indicated by the National Institute of Diabetes and Digestive and Kidney Diseases (NIDDK), diabetes duplicates your gamble of coronary illness and stroke. As well as observing and controlling your blood glucose, good dieting propensities and normal activity can assist with bringing down the gamble of hypertension and elevated cholesterol levels.
Assuming you smoke, consider stopping on the off chance that you're in danger of diabetes. Smoking builds your gamble of cardiovascular issues and confined blood stream. Your PCP can assist you with making a quit plan.

Absence of blood stream can ultimately influence your hands and feet, and cause torment while you're strolling. This is called discontinuous claudication.
The limited veins in your legs and feet may likewise bring on some issues in those areas. For instance, your feet might feel cold, or you might not be able to feel heat because of an absence of sensation.

This condition is known as fringe neuropathy, which is a kind of diabetic neuropathy that creates diminished uproar in the limits. It's especially perilous in light of the fact that it might keep you from seeing a physical issue or disease.
Diabetes additionally expands your gamble of creating contaminations or ulcers of the foot. Unfortunate blood stream and nerve harm improves the probability of having a foot or leg severed.

Assuming you have diabetes, it's important that you take great consideration of your feet and review them frequently.

Integumentary framework

Diabetes can likewise influence your skin, the biggest organ of your body. Alongside parchedness, your body's absence of dampness because of high glucose can make the skin on your feet dry and break.

It means quite a bit to dry your feet after washing or swimming totally. You can utilize oil jam or delicate creams, however try not to allow these regions to turn out to be excessively wet.

Sodden, warm overlap in the skin is powerless to parasitic, bacterial, or yeast diseases. These will generally foster in the accompanying regions:

- Among fingers and toes
- The crotch
- Armpits
- Corners of the mouth

Side effects incorporate redness, rankling, and irritation.

High-pressure spots under your foot can prompt calluses. These can become contaminated or foster ulcers. In the event that you really do get an ulcer, see a specialist quickly to bring down the gamble of losing your foot.

You may likewise be more inclined to:

- Bubbles
- Folliculitis (disease of the hair follicles)
- Eye sores
- Contaminated nails

Unmanaged diabetes can likewise prompt three skin conditions:

Eruptive xanthomatosis causes hard yellow knocks with a red ring.

Computerized sclerosis causes toughness, most frequently on the hands or feet.

Diabetic dermopathy can cause earthy colored patches on the skin. There's no reason to worry and no treatment is important.

These skin conditions generally clear up when glucose fixes.

Focal sensory system

Diabetes causes diabetic neuropathy, or harm to the nerves. This can influence your view of intensity, cold, and agony. It can likewise make you more powerless to injury.
The possibilities that you won't see these wounds and allow them to form into serious diseases or conditions increments, as well.

Diabetes can likewise prompt enlarged, broken veins in the eye, called diabetic retinopathy. This can harm your vision. It might try and prompt visual deficiency. Side effects of eye inconvenience can be gentle from the start, so it's vital to see your eye specialist routinely.

Conceptual framework

The changing chemicals during pregnancy can cause gestational diabetes and, thus, builds your gamble of hypertension. There are two kinds of hypertension conditions to keep an eye out for during pregnancy: toxemia and eclampsia.

By and large, gestational diabetes is effortlessly made due, and glucose levels get back to business as usual after the child is conceived. Side effects are like different sorts of diabetes however may likewise incorporate rehashed contaminations influencing the vagina and bladder.
On the off chance that you foster gestational diabetes, your child might have a higher birth weight. This can make conveyance more convoluted. You're additionally at an expanded gamble of creating type 2 diabetes quite a while following your child's conveyance.

Indications of type 2 diabetes

The side effects of type 2 diabetes change from one individual to another. They can foster gradually over numerous years and may be gentle to such an extent that you don't see them.

- Incessant pee
- Polyuria, or inordinate pee, is one of the 3 P's of diabetes.

Your kidneys in the long run can't stay aware of the additional glucose in your circulatory system. A portion of the glucose winds up in your pee and attracts more water. This prompts more regular pee.
Grown-ups normally produce 1 to 2 liters of pee each day (a liter is about a quart). Polyuria is characterized as multiple liters each day.

Outrageous thirst

Unreasonable thirst, or polydipsia, is much of the time a consequence of successive pee. Your body urges you to supplant lost liquids by causing you to feel parched.

Obviously, everybody gets parched now and then. Outrageous thirst is strange and relentless, regardless of how frequently you renew.

Expanded hunger
Unnecessary yearning is called polyphagia.

In the event that you have type 2 diabetes, your body struggles with transforming glucose into energy. This causes you to feel hungry. Eating presents significantly more sugar that can't be handled, and it doesn't mitigate hunger.

1. Foggy vision
2. Diabetes builds your gamble of a few eye conditions,, including:
    - Diabetic retinopathy
    - Waterfalls
    - Open-point glaucoma

The expanded glucose from diabetes can harm veins, remembering those for the eye, prompting foggy vision.

Exhaustion

Exhaustion can be a psychological or actual sluggishness that doesn't improve with rest. There are many reasons for exhaustion. It's a troublesome side effect to explore, however a recent report reasoned that individuals with type 2 diabetes might encounter weakness because of changes among high and low glucose levels.

Slow-mending wounds

Assuming you have type 2 diabetes, normal cuts and scratches can take more time to mend. Wounds on your feet are normal and barely noticeable. Slow recuperating foot ulcers happen because of unfortunate blood supply as well as harm to the nerves liable for bloodstream to the feet.

A recent report showed that diabetic foot ulcers don't prepare the resistant cells required for legitimate irritation and mending.

High glucose can harm the veins that supply supplements to your nerves. At the point when your nerves don't get sufficient oxygen and supplements, they can't work as expected.

This is called **diabetic neuropathy** and is most normal in your limits.

Unexplained weight reduction

Insulin obstruction makes glucose develop in the circulatory system as opposed to being transformed into energy. This can make your body consume other energy sources, similar to muscle or fat tissue.

Your weight could normally change a bit. An unexplained loss of no less than 5% of your body weight is by and large concurred as a need to converse with your medical care proficient.

Incessant contaminations

Notwithstanding nerve harm and a debilitated resistant framework, unfortunate blood flow likewise expands the possibility of fostering contamination in individuals with diabetes. Having more sugar in your blood and tissues permits diseases to spread quicker.

Individuals with diabetes normally foster diseases of the:

- Ear, nose, and throat
- Kidney
- Bladder
- Feet

- Areas of obscured skin, like the armpits or neck

Acanthosis nigricans is a skin condition that can be a side effect of diabetes. It shows up as dim groups of skin that might have a smooth surface.
This is most normal in body overlays like your armpits, neck, and crotch, however can likewise happen somewhere else.

1. Side effects of type 2 diabetes in men While the side effects above can happen in anybody with type 2 diabetes, the accompanying side effects are well defined for men, or people who are appointed male upon entering the world:Men with diabetes have lower levels of testosterone, which a recent report connected to a diminished sex drive.A survey of examinations distributed in 2017 observed that the greater part of men with diabetes are impacted by ED.A few men might encounter retrograde discharge as a side effect of diabetes, as indicated by research.The lower testosterone levels saw in men with diabetes may likewise add to decreased bulk.

2. Side effects of type 2 diabetes in ladiesType 2 diabetes additionally may give side effects well defined for ladies, for example,UTIs are more normal in ladies and are more normal and extreme in those with type 2 diabetes, as per a survey of exploration distributed in 2015.Raised glucose levels permit yeast creatures to develop all the more effectively, prompting a higher opportunity of contamination.
   Type 2 diabetes doesn't explicitly make it more hard to consider, however polycystic ovary condition (PCOS) can. Creating PCOS has been connected to insulin obstruction, and PCOS has been displayed to expand the gamble of type 2 diabetes, as indicated by the CDC,.

Are there side effects of prediabetes 2?
Prediabetes is a medical issue where your glucose is higher than it should be, however it's not sufficiently high for a specialist to determine you have type 2 diabetes.

More than 1 out of 3. American grown-ups have prediabetes, numerous without knowing it. There are typically no side effects of prediabetes, however there are steps you can take to assist with forestalling creating it:

Losing overabundance weight and keeping a moderate weight

Practicing as frequently as could really be expected

Changing your eating regimen, zeroing in on supplement rich, adjusted eating plan

Drinking water rather than low-supplement refreshments such sweet beverages

There are numerous side effects that you might insight into assuming you have type 2 diabetes. They can be inconspicuous and could foster throughout quite a while.

Type 2 diabetes can be eased back or even forestalled. In the event that you accept you might be encountering side effects of diabetes, examine your interests with a characteristic ways of helping your insulin

Part two:Type 1 Diabetes

Chapter five:

Another comprehension of Type 1 Diabetes

Type 1 Diabetes is significantly less normal than type 2, it is generally analyzed in adolescence and is constantly treated with insulin has its previous names, youth beginning diabetes and insulin-subordinate diabetes.
Dissimilar to individuals with type 2 diabetes, type one in every case needs to take insulin. Yet, they can utilize diet and way of life changes to downplay portions and diminish the gamble of confusions. We likewise have another comprehension of the principal reasons for type 1 diabetes starting when the body's resistant framework goes after the insulin-delivering cells of the pancreas. As you will see, new exploration has uncovered what seems to start that demeanor and what can assist with forestalling it.

Type 1 diabetes once known as adolescent diabetes or insulin-subordinate diabetes is a persistent condition. In this condition, the pancreas makes next to zero insulin to stop insulin is a chemical that the body uses to permit sugar (glucose) to enter cells to create energy.

Various variables, for example, hereditary qualities and some infections, may cause type 1 diabetes. I really do think type 1 diabetes generally shows up during youth or pre-adulthood, it can foster in grown-ups. Indeed, even after a great deal of examination, type 1 diabetes has no solution for strep treatment and is coordinated towards dealing with how much sugar in the blood utilizes insulin, diet and way of life to forestall difficulties.

Side effects

Type 1 diabetes side effects can show up out of nowhere and may include:
-Feeling more testing than expected.
-Peeing a ton.
-Bed-wetting in kids who have never worked the bed during the evening.
-Shedding pounds almost too easily.
-Feeling peevish or having other state of mind changes.
-Feeling drained and feeble.
-Having hazy vision.

Causes

The specific reason for type 1 diabetes is obscure. Typically the body's own resistant framework which ordinarily battles unsafe microbes and infections obliterates the insulin-delivering (islet) cells in the pancreas.
Other potential causes incorporate;
-Hereditary qualities.
-Openness to invulnerable and other ecological variables.
Job of Insulin and Glucose for a more grounded Muscles and Energy stockpiling

Chapter six

The major job of insulin and Glucose for a stronger Muscles and Energy storage

The job of Insulin

When an enormous number of islets cells are obliterated, the body creates practically no insulin. Insulin is a chemical that comes from an organ behind and underneath the stomach (pancreas).
-The pancreas places insulin into the circulatory system.
-Insulin goes through the body permitting sugar to enter the cells.
-Insulin brings down how much sugar is in the circulation system.
-As the glucose level drops, the pancreas places less insulin into the circulation system.

The job of glucose

Glucose-a sugar-is a primary wellspring of energy that makes muscles and different tissues.
-Glucose comes from two significant sources: food and the liver.
-Sugar is retained into the circulation system, where it enters cells with the insulin.
-The liver stores glucose as glycogen.
-At the point when glucose levels are low, for example, when you haven't eaten in some time, the liver separates the put away glycogen into glucose. This keeps glucose level inside a normal reach.

In type 1 diabetes, there's no insulin to give glucose access to the cells. As a result of this sugar develops in the circulation system. This can cause hazardous entanglements

Entanglements

Extra time, type 1 diabetes entanglements can influence significant organs in the body. These organs incorporate the heart, veins, Nerves, eyes and kidneys. Having a typical glucose level can bring down the gamble of numerous inconveniences.

Diabetes intricacies can prompt handicaps or even undermine your life.

-Heart and veins.

Diabetes builds the gamble of certain issues with the heart and veins. These incorporate coronary corridor infections like chest pain(angina), cardiovascular failure, stroke, restricting of the courses (atherosclerosis) and hypertension.

-Nerve harm (neuropathy)

An excessive amount of sugar in the blood can destroy the walls of the minuscule veins (vessels) that feed the nerves. This is particularly evident in the legs. This can cause shivering, deadness, consuming or torment. This typically starts at the tips of the toes or fingers and spreads upwards. Early control of glucose can make you lose all feeling in the impacted names after some time.

-Kidney harm (nephropathy)

The kidney has a great many minuscule veins that hold squander back from entering the blood. Diabetes can harm this framework. extreme harm can prompt kidney disappointment or end stage kidney sickness that can't be turned around.

-Skin and mouth conditions

Diabetes might leave you more inclined to contaminations of the mouth and skin. This incorporates bacteria and parasitics.

Chapter seven

Insulin Resistance: The flood peculiarity

The fact that we can't survive without insulin is a fundamental chemical. What occurs, in any case, when our tissues experience difficulty answering it? That is insulin obstruction.
Insulin obstruction is an extremely normal condition that frequently goes with heftiness or a conclusion of pre-diabetes, type 2 diabetes, polycystic ovary disorder (PCOS), cardiovascular illness, and other metabolic circumstances like hypertension and non-alcoholic greasy liver sickness.

Have you been informed you have insulin obstruction? You're in good company.

Based on NHANES 2011-2016 information, the predominance of the insulin opposition condition (AKA metabolic disorder) in the United States is 35%. However the general rate has been genuinely steady since the NHANES 2003-2006 information was delivered, the predominance of metabolic disorder among youthful grown-ups, Hispanic people, and Asian people has shown a measurably huge increment.

At the point when we take a gander at individuals with heftiness, the numbers deteriorate. Insulin obstruction can be viewed as in up to 44% of teenagers and 70% of ladies with weight. Among grown-ups with type 2 diabetes, the commonness of insulin obstruction ascends to more than 80%.
The fact that they have it makes numerous people with the condition ignorant.
Additionally concerning? Insulin obstruction is being connected to an expanded gamble of certain malignant growths, Alzheimer's sickness, emotional wellness problems, and other constant circumstances.

What is insulin obstruction?

Insulin obstruction is when cells in your body don't answer successfully to the chemical insulin that is circling in your body. This makes the pancreas emit significantly a greater amount of this significant chemical with an end goal to keep your glucose from ascending excessively high.

Insulin plays many parts. Its essential job is to keep our blood glucose levels in an exceptionally close reach — called blood glucose homeostasis. That is on the grounds that both too high and too low blood glucose levels are perilous and harming to the body. At the point when glucose levels rise, more insulin is emitted. At the point when glucose levels fall, less insulin is discharged. Since more significant levels of insulin have been related with various persistent medical issues, it's a good idea that keeping insulin in a lower physiologic reach might be better for your drawn out wellbeing.

Insulin likewise empowers glucose to be utilized by cells for fuel or put away as glycogen in muscle and liver cells. Falling degrees of insulin let the liver know when to make more glucose (gluconeogenesis) and rising insulin levels let the liver know when to stop.

One more significant job is insulin's guideline of fat stockpiling. At the point when insulin levels are high, it invigorates fat cells to take up glucose and transform it into fat (lipogenesis). Then, when insulin is low, it empowers the body to remove the fat from stockpiling and use it for energy.

For somebody who is metabolically solid, this interaction works consistently to guarantee a steady inventory of fuel for the body. The issue emerges when we are not metabolically sound, which a few scientists gauge might be the situation for as numerous as 88% of Americans.

The other significant piece of understanding insulin opposition is a condition that habitually concurs with it called hyperinsulinemia. At the point when our bodies are presented to a tenacious stockpile of glucose, insulin is continually emitted and remains constantly high hyperinsulinemia.

Hyperinsulinemia is logical both a reason and an impact of insulin opposition.

For what reason does insulin obstruction occur?

Hereditary gamble factors, natural gamble variables, and way of life factors have all been found to add to the advancement of insulin obstruction.

While certain individuals might be hereditarily bound to foster insulin obstruction, the greatest effect has maybe come from the adjustment of our food climate in ongoing many years. More noteworthy accessibility of modest, energy-thick food and beverages might have driven entire populaces to take on an unfortunate way of life, portrayed by utilization of elevated degrees of sugar and other refined starches. These basic carbs are changed over into a lot of glucose that we may not require for energy, frequently bringing about quite a bit of it being put away in our phones or put away as fat.

Researchers have clarified numerous components and pathways that add to the advancement of insulin opposition. Strangely, despite the fact that we frequently consider insulin opposition as far as the impact of insulin on glucose digestion, one of the significant causes is really disarranged unsaturated fat digestion.

Logical proof recommends that unsaturated fats improperly amass in muscle and liver which then slows down their cells' capacity to answer insulin and take up glucose. One of the primary inquiries, thusly, is how do abundance of unsaturated fats attack muscle and liver cells?

One system includes the over-utilization of sugar, particularly fructose, and especially in the setting of abundance caloric admission. Through different pathways that are past the extent of this article, this is remembered to prompt exorbitant creation of fat in the liver, which then prompts expanded insulin opposition.

The equivalent is logically valid for a high starch, high fat eating routine in the setting of overabundant calories. A few examinations propose that explicitly immersed fat more so than MUFAs and PUFAs is the guilty party that causes insulin obstruction.

Regardless, it is essential to take note of that none of those reviews remembered soaked fats for the setting of a low-carb diet. Certifiable investigations of low-carb slims down without any limitations on soaked fat have tracked down enhancements and even standardization of insulin obstruction markers. This

recommends that the issue may not be immersed fat itself, yet rather the mix of soaked fats and a high measure of starches.
Also, as we audit in our proof put together with respect to soaked fat, it isn't precise to allude to immersed fat as a certain something. Immersed fat from cakes, treats, and other prepared products could meaningfully affect the body than additional normally happening soaked fats in meat and dairy.

At long last, a basic idea to comprehend is that raised insulin itself might deteriorate insulin opposition. This makes an endless loop of insulin opposition and hyperinsulinemia likely exacerbated by progressing caloric overabundance and weight gain.

Side effects of insulin opposition

Insulin opposition has no undeniable side effects of infirmity.

The fundamental indication of the condition in many individuals preceding being determined to have pre-diabetes or out and out type 2 diabetes is expanding stomach fat, albeit not every person will know about this.

A predominant hypothesis of how insulin opposition deteriorates is that we each have an edge level of fat that can be put away in our fat cells and when this is surpassed, our body begins putting away fat in not so great spots — particularly around the organs in our mid-region (like the liver and the pancreas) and in our stomach pit. This is called instinctive fat and when this fat begins expanding, it is a certain indication of insulin obstruction.
Other unpretentious indications of insulin obstruction in certain individuals are dull, dry patches of skin on the crotch, armpits, or back of the neck, known as acanthosis nigricans. Skin labels little plump developments frequently on the neck or armpits can likewise be an indication of insulin obstruction in certain individuals, which is remembered to happen on the grounds that insulin is a trigger of cell development.

Other than those side effects, a great many people with early insulin obstruction feel fine. It is just as blood glucose at long last begins to rise that different side effects of high glucose and type 2 diabetes might start to show, like regular pee, unnecessary thirst, weariness, and extreme yearning.

It is critical to comprehend that insulin levels climb increasingly high trying to monitor blood glucose. For some time, this worked. However, ultimately the pancreatic beta cells that make insulin dynamically come up short, to the place where insulin levels are presently not sufficiently high to control blood glucose, so blood glucose levels begin to rise. This may not occur until late in the sickness cycle.

When somebody is determined to have type 2 diabetes, they have presumably had insulin opposition or persistent hyperinsulinemia for various years, maybe much over 10 years.

Conditions related with insulin opposition

The accompanying medical issue are related with insulin opposition:

- Corpulence — Insulin obstruction is related with high insulin levels that might prompt expanded body weight and stoutness; heftiness thus prompts expanded insulin opposition, in this way making an endless loop.

- Pregnancy — Many ladies give indications of insulin obstruction during pregnancy, particularly in the third trimester. This is accepted to be a developmental transformation to give adequate glucose to the quickly developing embryo. Nonetheless, in certain individuals, this can prompt gestational diabetes and hypertension. Defenders of the low-carb way of life accept this is an ideal illustration of how an ordinary transformation intended to assist with guaranteeing sound pregnancy makes us more powerless to metabolic sickness with regards to a cutting edge diet with food sources high in refined starches, fats and sugars.

- Metabolic disorder — This portrays an assortment of qualities that are tracked down in individuals with insulin opposition. There are various definitions for metabolic conditions that generally incorporate a raised fasting blood glucose level, hypertension, raised fatty substances and decreased HDL cholesterol, and expanded midsection boundary.

- Pre-diabetes — Insulin opposition is related to pre-diabetes. This is in which blood glucose levels are higher than ordinary yet not yet sufficiently high for a determination of type 2 diabetes. The World Health Organization characterizes pre-diabetes as a fasting glucose of 110 - 125 mg/dL (6.1 - 6.9 mmol/L) or a 2-hour glucose of 140 - 200 mg/dL (7.8 - 11.1 mmol/L), as estimated after a normalized 75-gram oral glucose challenge.The US and a few different nations utilize an alternate meaning of FBG 100 - 125 mg/dL (5.7 - 6.9 mmol/L) or HbA1c 5.7 - 6.4% (39 - 46 mmol/mol). Since a finding of pre-diabetes relies upon a raised blood glucose level, it infers that insulin levels have been persistently raised for quite a while before the conclusion.

- Polycystic ovary condition (PCOS) — Polycystic ovary condition (PCOS) is a typical metabolic problem influencing up to 10% of ladies of childbearing age. It's a main source of fruitlessness, and builds the gamble of creating type 2 diabetes in later life. Ladies with PCOS will generally have raised degrees of male chemicals, sporadic or missing feminine periods, and growths on their ovaries, as well as insulin obstruction. Other normal side effects are stoutness, skin break out, male-design balding, and overabundance of facial and body hair.

Step by step instructions to switch PCOS with low carb
GUIDE Polycystic ovary disorder (PCOS) is normal, influencing up to 10% of ladies of childbearing age. Past feminine issues and other actual side effects, it's a main source of fruitlessness.
Non-Alcoholic Fatty Liver Disease — Called NAFLD, this is where there is a lot of fat put away in the liver. It very well might be the consequence of persistently high insulin levels and it might add to insulin obstruction. While it is more normal in people with heftiness, metabolic disorder, and type 2 diabetes, it has been viewed as related with insulin opposition and hyperinsulinemia in lean people with typical glucose resistance. Certain individuals with NAFLD proceed to foster liver issues, like aggravation, scarring, and cirrhosis as well as liver disappointment.

- Disease — Insulin opposition is related with an expansion in chance of colorectal malignant growth, endometrial malignant growth, pancreatic malignant growth, and bosom disease. It isn't evident whether it is the insulin opposition itself or its relationship to other gamble factors, for example, heftiness and high blood glucose, that adds to the expanded disease risk. Nonetheless, constantly elevated degrees of insulin might advance disease development and that diminishing insulin levels might slow malignant growth development, albeit more information is required around here to make firm determinations.

- Cardiovascular illness (CVD) — Insulin opposition and hyperinsulinemia are related with expanded takes a chance for cardiovascular sickness, to a limited extent since they are so firmly connected with other CVD risk factors like stoutness and hypertension. A few examinations propose, nonetheless, that insulin opposition is a free gamble factor for coronary illness. There are various hypotheses about why hyperinsulinemia could set off moderate coronary illness. The greater part of them is based on expanded constant irritation and oxidation as well as immediate vascular harm.

- Alzheimer's sickness — Recent proof proposes that Alzheimer's infection could likewise be connected to insulin obstruction. Concentrates on showing that those with diabetes are 60% bound to foster dementia. Another review shows an expanded predominance of mind degeneration in those with diabetes.Albeit the specific instrument isn't demonstrated, the hypothesis is that synapses become insulin safe and afterward can't utilize glucose proficiently for fuel, subsequently leaving the cells starving for energy. The outcome is possible movement to Alzheimer's sickness.

- Versatile insulin obstruction — Eating extremely low-carb slims down has been related with the improvement of insulin opposition. Nonetheless, some guess that this is a versatile physiologic reaction, and hence the name versatile or physiologic insulin opposition.

While this isn't demonstrated, we can estimate that assuming we quit eating sugar or carbs, how much glucose in our blood will fall, essentially somewhat. Our body will ensure, nonetheless, that our mind gets the glucose it needs by not sending as much glucose to the liver, fat cells or muscle cells (in this way those tissues and cells show up "insulin safe"). The cerebrum can then involve a mix of glucose and ketones as fuel.The muscle and liver cells rather use ketones solely for fuel. Since this kind of insulin opposition happens with low instead of elevated degrees of coursing insulin, it isn't felt to address a similar perilous condition as customary insulin obstruction and may really be something to be thankful for.

Furthermore, one concentrate in solid workers plainly showed further developed liver insulin responsiveness with a day and a half of fasting contrasted with 12 hours, bringing about lower generally glucose and insulin levels, all regardless of what might be thought of "fringe insulin opposition." The creators reasoned that the liver insulin awareness makes this a sound reaction, rather than hepatic insulin obstruction in the pathologic form of insulin opposition.

Diagnosing insulin opposition

How can you say whether you have insulin opposition? What tests could you at any point have that will affirm the conclusion?

Sadly, insulin obstruction is seldom analyzed in most clinical practices. It's not on the grounds that it isn't broadly predominant in the public arena, but since specialists don't for the most part arrange the tests for it.

All things being equal, specialists all the more frequently request the standard tests for diabetes that action glucose levels: fasting blood glucose and hemoglobin A1c. In any case, when these are raised, insulin levels have likely been high for a really long time, on the off chance that not many years.

Nonetheless, know that not all wellbeing frameworks give inclusion to insulin levels and you might need to pay the full expense yourself.

Soaked and trans fats, which can support insulin obstruction. These come mostly from creature sources, like meats and cheddar, as well as food sources broiled in somewhat hydrogenated oils. Improved drinks, similar to pop, natural product drinks, chilled teas, and nutrient water, which can make you put on weight.

Section three: Type 2 Diabetes-Sugar

Chapter Eight

Type 2 Diabetes-Medical Complications

Type 2 diabetes mellitus comprises a variety of dysfunctions portrayed by hyperglycemia and coming about because of the blend of protection from insulin activity, insufficient insulin discharge, and over the top or unseemly glucagon emission. Inadequately controlled type 2 diabetes is related with a variety of microvascular, macrovascular, and neuropathic inconveniences.

Microvascular complexities of diabetes incorporate retinal, renal, and perhaps neuropathic illness. Macrovascular complexities incorporate coronary vein and fringe vascular illness. Diabetic neuropathy influences autonomic and fringe nerves. (See Pathophysiology and Presentation.)

Dissimilar to patients with type 1 diabetes mellitus, patients with type 2 are not actually reliant upon insulin forever. This differentiation was the reason for the more established terms for types 1 and 2, insulin subordinate and non-insulin subordinate diabetes.

Nonetheless, numerous patients with type 2 diabetes are at last treated with insulin. Since they hold the capacity to emit some endogenous insulin, they are considered to require insulin yet not to rely upon insulin. By the way, given the potential for disarray because of grouping in light of treatment as opposed to etiology, the more seasoned terms have been abandoned.Another more established term for type 2 diabetes mellitus was grown-up beginning diabetes. Right now, in light of the pestilence of weight and idleness in kids, type 2 diabetes mellitus is happening at increasingly young ages. Despite the fact that type 2 diabetes mellitus commonly influences people more seasoned than 40 years, it has been analyzed in kids as youthful as 2 years old who have a family background of diabetes. In numerous networks,

type 2 diabetes presently dwarfs type 1 among youngsters with recently analyzed diabetes. (See Epidemiology.)
Diabetes mellitus is an ongoing sickness that requires long haul clinical thoughtfulness regarding limiting the improvement of its overwhelming entanglements and to oversee them when they do happen. It is an excessively costly sickness; in the United States in 2012, the immediate and backhanded expenses of analyzed diabetes were assessed to be $245 billion; individuals with analyzed diabetes had normal clinical consumptions 2.3 times those of individuals without diabetes.

Pathophysiology

Type 2 diabetes is portrayed by a blend of fringe insulin obstruction and lacking insulin discharge by pancreatic beta cells. Insulin obstruction, which has been ascribed to raised degrees of free unsaturated fats and proinflammatory cytokines in plasma, prompts diminished glucose transport into muscle cells, raised hepatic glucose creation, and expanded breakdown of fat.
A job for overabundance glucagon can't be undervalued; for sure, type 2 diabetes is an islet paracrine pathway in which the corresponding connection between the glucagon-discharging alpha cell and the insulin-emitting beta cell is lost, prompting hyperglucagonemia and subsequently the ensuing hyperglycemia.
For type 2 diabetes mellitus to happen, both insulin opposition and lacking insulin emission should exist. For instance, all overweight people have insulin obstruction, yet diabetes grows just in the individuals who can't increment insulin emission adequately to make up for their insulin opposition. Their insulin fixations might be high, yet improperly low for the degree of glycemia.
A worked on plot for the pathophysiology of unusual glucose digestion in type 2 diabetes mellitus is portrayed in the picture underneath.

Beta-cell brokenness

Beta-cell brokenness is a central point across the range of prediabetes to diabetes. An investigation of large youths by Bacha et al affirms what is progressively being focused on in grown-ups too: Beta-cell brokenness grows right off the bat in the pathologic cycle and doesn't be guaranteed to follow the phase of insulin opposition. Solitary spotlight on insulin opposition as the "most important thing in the world" is slowly moving, and ideally better treatment choices that address the beta-cell pathology will arise for early treatment.

Genomic factors

Vast affiliation investigations of single-nucleotide polymorphisms (SNPs) have recognized various hereditary variations that are related with beta-cell capability and insulin opposition. A portion of these SNPs seem to build the gamble for type 2 diabetes. More than 40 autonomous loci exhibiting a relationship with an expanded gamble for type 2 diabetes have been shown. A subset of the most intense are shared underneath;

- Diminished beta-cell responsiveness, prompting weakened insulin handling and diminished insulinemission (TCF7L2)
- Brought down early glucose-animated insulin discharge (MTNR1B, FADS1, DGKB, GCK)
- Adjusted digestion of unsaturated fats (FADS1)
- Dysregulation of fat digestion (PPARG)
- Restraint of serum glucose discharge (KCNJ11)
- Expanded adiposity and insulin opposition (FTO and IGF2BP2)
- Control of the improvement of pancreatic designs, including beta-islet cells (HHEX)
- Transport of zinc into the beta-islet cells, which impacts the creation and emission of insulin (SLC30A8)
- Endurance and capability of beta-islet cells (WFS1)

Powerlessness to type 2 diabetes may likewise be impacted by hereditary variations including incretin chemicals, which are let out of endocrine cells in the stomach and animate insulin emission in light of absorption of food. For instance, diminished beta-cell capability has been related with a variation in the quality that codes for the receptor of gastric inhibitory polypeptide (GIPR).

The high versatility bunch A1 (HMGA1) protein is a critical controller of the insulin receptor quality (INSR). Utilitarian variations of the HMGA1 quality are related with an expanded gamble of diabetes.

Amino corrosive digestion

Amino corrosive digestion might assume a critical part right off the bat in the improvement of type 2 diabetes. Wang et al revealed that the gamble of future diabetes was somewhere around 4-crease higher in normoglycemic people with high fasting plasma convergences of 3 amino acids (isoleucine, phenylalanine, and tyrosine). Convergences of these amino acids were raised as long as 12 years preceding the beginning of diabetes. In this review, amino acids, amines, and other polar metabolites were profiled utilizing fluid chromatography coupled mass spectrometry.

Diabetes complexities

Albeit the pathophysiology of the sickness contrasts between the sorts of diabetes, the vast majority of the confusions, including microvascular, macrovascular, and neuropathic, are comparative no matter what the kind of diabetes. Hyperglycemia has all the earmarks of being the determinant of microvascular and metabolic difficulties. Macrovascular sickness might be less connected with glycemia.

Telomere weakening might be a marker related with presence and the quantity of diabetic difficulties. Whether it is a reason or a result of diabetes is not yet clear.

Cardiovascular gamble

Cardiovascular gamble in individuals with diabetes is connected to some degree to insulin obstruction, with the accompanying corresponding lipid irregularities:

- Raised degrees of little, thick low-thickness lipoprotein (LDL) cholesterol particles

- Low degrees of high-thickness lipoprotein (HDL) cholesterol

- Raised degrees of fatty substance rich leftover lipoproteins

- Thrombotic irregularities (ie, raised type-1 plasminogen activator inhibitor [PAI-1], raised fibrinogen) and hypertension are additionally involved. Other regular atherosclerotic gamble factors (eg, family ancestry, smoking, raised LDL cholesterol) likewise influence cardiovascular gamble.

Etiology

The etiology of type 2 diabetes mellitus seems to include complex communications among ecological and hereditary variables. Probably, the sickness is created when a diabetogenic way of life (ie, over the top caloric admission, insufficient caloric use, stoutness) is superimposed on a vulnerable genotype.

The weight record (BMI) at which overabundance weight increments risk for diabetes shifts with various racial gatherings. For instance, contrasted and people of European family, people of Asian lineage are at expanded risk for diabetes at lower levels of overweight. Hypertension and prehypertension are related with a more serious gamble of creating diabetes in whites than in African Americans.

Also, an in utero climate bringing about low birth weight might incline a few people toward fostering kind 2 diabetes mellitus. Baby weight speed has a little, circuitous impact on grown-up insulin obstruction, and this is principally intervened through its impact on BMI and midsection boundary.

Roughly 90% of people with type 2 diabetes mellitus are overweight or have obesity.However, a huge, populace based, planned study has shown that an energy-thick eating routine might be a gamble factor for the improvement of diabetes that is free of pattern stoutness.

A concentrate by Cameron et al showed that in the United States somewhere in the range of 2013 and 2016, weight was liable for the improvement of new-beginning diabetes in 41% of grown-ups. The most noteworthy inferable pace of stoutness related diabetes was among non-Hispanic White ladies (53%); non-Hispanic Black men exhibited the least rate, with the inferable part being 30%.

A few examinations propose that natural poisons might assume a part in the turn of events and movement of type 2 diabetes mellitus. An organized and arranged stage is expected to

completely investigate the diabetes-instigating capability of natural contaminations.
Auxiliary diabetes might happen in patients taking glucocorticoids or when patients have conditions that irritate the activities of insulin (eg, Cushing disorder, acromegaly, pheochromocytoma).

A concentrate by Pauza et al recommended that glucagon-like peptide-1 (GLP-1) is related with the connection among diabetes and hypertension. The specialists observed that GLP-1 receptors are communicated on the carotid body and, working with rodents, discovered that diminished articulation of these receptors "is connected to thoughtful hyperactivity in rodents with cardiometabolic sickness." Thus, the examination shows that GLP-1 not just has its known impact in glucose control (by animating insulin discharge) yet is related with pulse control too.

Significant gamble factors
The significant gamble factors for type 2 diabetes mellitus are the accompanying:

- Age more prominent than 45 years (however, as verified above, type 2 diabetes mellitus is happening with expanding recurrence in youthful people)
- Weight more prominent than 120% of beneficial body weight
- Family background of type 2 diabetes in a first-degree relative (eg, parent or kin)
- Hispanic, Native American, African American, Asian American, or Pacific Islander plummet
- History of past impeded glucose resilience (IGT) or debilitated fasting glucose (IFG)
- Hypertension (>140/90 mm Hg) or dyslipidemia (HDL cholesterol level < 40 mg/dL or fatty substance level >150 mg/dL)

History of gestational diabetes mellitus or of conveying a child with a birth weight of more than 9 lb

Polycystic ovarian condition (which brings about insulin opposition)

Hereditary impacts

The hereditary qualities of type 2 diabetes are complicated and not totally perceived. Proof backings the contribution of various qualities in pancreatic beta-cell disappointment and insulin opposition.

Vast affiliation studies have recognized many normal hereditary variations related with expanded risk for type 2 diabetes.Of the variations hitherto found, the one with the most grounded impact on powerlessness is the record factor 7-like 2 (TCF7L2) quality. (For more data, see Type 2 Diabetes and TCF7L2.)

Distinguished hereditary variations represent just around 10% of the heritable part of most sort 2 diabetes. A global exploration consortium found that utilization of a 40-SNP hereditary gamble score works on the capacity to make a surmised 8-year risk expectation for diabetes past that which is reachable when just normal clinical diabetes risk factors are utilized. Additionally, the prescient capacity is better in more youthful people (in whom early preventive procedures could defer diabetes beginning) than in those more seasoned than 50 years.

A few types of diabetes have a reasonable relationship with hereditary deformities. The condition generally known as development beginning diabetes of youth (MODY), which is currently perceived to be various deformities in beta-cell capability, represents 2-5% of people with type 2 diabetes who present early in life and have a mild illness. The characteristic is autosomal predominant and can be evaluated through business research centers.

Until now, 11 MODY subtypes have been recognized, including changes in the accompanying qualities [60, 61] :

- ☐ HNF-4-alpha
- ☐ Glucokinase quality
- ☐ HNF-1-alpha
- ☐ IPF-1
- ☐ HNF-1-beta
- ☐ NEUROD1
- ☐ KLF11 [62]

- ☐ CEL [63]
- ☐ PAX4 [64]
- ☐ INS
- ☐ BLK [65]

The greater part of the MODY subtypes are related with diabetes just; in any case, MODY type 5 is known to be related with renal pimples, and MODY type 8 is related with exocrine pancreatic brokenness. Various variations in mitochondrial deoxyribonucleic corrosive (DNA) have been proposed as an etiologic element for a small level of patients with type 2 diabetes. Two explicit point transformations and a few erasures and duplications in the mitochondrial genome can cause type 2 diabetes and sensorineural hearing misfortune.

Diabetes can likewise be found in more extreme mitochondrial issues like Kearns-Sayre disorder and mitochondrial encephalomyopathy, lactic acidosis, and stroke like episode (MELAS). Mitochondrial types of diabetes mellitus ought to be thought about when diabetes happens related to hearing misfortune, myopathy, seizure jumble, strokelike episodes, retinitis pigmentosa, outside ophthalmoplegia, or waterfalls. These discoveries are of specific importance assuming that there is proof of maternal legacy.

A meta-investigation of two examinations demonstrated that a hereditarily related low birth weight builds a singular's gamble for creating type 2 diabetes. The report found that for every one-point expansion in a person's hereditary gamble score for low birth weight, the sort 2 diabetes risk rose by 6%.

Melancholy

Gathering proof recommends that downturn is a critical gamble factor for creating type 2 diabetes. Skillet et al observed that the overall gamble was 1.17 in ladies with discouraged mind-set and 1.25 in ladies utilizing antidepressants. Energizer use might be a marker of more extreme, ongoing, or repetitive sadness, or stimulant use itself might increase diabetes risk, conceivably by changing glucose homeostasis or advancing weight gain.

Thus, type 2 diabetes has been distinguished as a gamble factor for the improvement of gloom. Burdensome side effects and significant burdensome issues are two times as pervasive in patients with type 2 diabetes as in everyone.

Schizophrenia

Schizophrenia has been connected to the gamble for type 2 diabetes. Useless flagging including protein kinase B (Akt) is a potential system for schizophrenia; additionally, gained Akt surrenders are related with debilitated guidelines of blood glucose and diabetes, which is overrepresented in first-episode, drug guileless patients with schizophrenia. Furthermore, second-age antipsychotics are related with more serious gamble for type-2 diabetes.

Metabolic Syndrome

Metabolic condition is an assortment of hazard factors that increase the possibility of coronary illness, stroke, and diabetes. Shedding pounds, exercise, and dietary changes can help forestall or turn around metabolic disorder.

What is metabolic disorder?

Metabolic disorder is an assortment of coronary illness risk factors that increment your possibility creating coronary illness, stroke, and diabetes. The condition is additionally realized by different names including Syndrome X, insulin opposition disorder, and dysmetabolic condition. As per a public wellbeing overview, more than 1 out of 5 Americans has metabolic disorder. The quantity of individuals with metabolic disorder increments with age, influencing over 40% of individuals in their 60s and 70s.

Who regularly has metabolic disorder?

Individuals with focal heftiness (expanded fat in the midsection/abdomen).

Individuals with diabetes mellitus or a solid family background of diabetes mellitus.

Individuals with other clinical elements of "insulin obstruction" including skin changes of acanthosis nigricans ("obscured skin" on the rear of the neck or underarms) or skin labels (typically on the neck).

Certain ethnic foundations are at a higher gamble of creating metabolic conditions.

As you become older, your gamble of creating metabolic disorder increases.

Side effects AND CAUSES

What causes metabolic disorder?

The specific reason for metabolic disorder isn't known. Many highlights of the metabolic condition are related to "insulin obstruction." Insulin opposition implies that the body doesn't utilize insulin effectively to bring down glucose and fatty oil levels. A mix of hereditary and way of life variables might bring about insulin opposition. Way of life factors incorporate dietary propensities, movement and maybe hindered rest designs (like rest apnea).

What are the side effects of metabolic condition?

Ordinarily, there are no quick actual side effects. Clinical issues related with metabolic disorder fosters after some time. Assuming that you are uncertain, assuming you have a metabolic condition, see your medical services supplier.The individual will actually want to make the finding by acquiring the important tests, including circulatory strain, lipid profile (fatty oils and HDL) and blood glucose.

Determination AND TESTS

How is metabolic disorder analyzed?

You are determined to have metabolic condition on the off chance that you have at least three of the accompanying:

A waistline of 40 inches or something else for men and 35 inches or something else for ladies (estimated across the midsection)

A pulse of 130/85 mm Hg or higher or are taking circulatory strain drugs

A fatty oil level over 150 mg/dl

A fasting blood glucose (sugar) level more noteworthy than 100 mg/dl or are taking glucose-bringing down drugs

A high thickness lipoprotein level (HDL) under 40 mg/dl (men) or under 50 mg/dl (ladies).

Anticipation

How would I forestall or switch metabolic disorder?

Since actual dormancy and overabundance weight are the vitally basic supporters of the improvement of metabolic disorder, working out, practicing good eating habits and, assuming you have overweight or heftiness, making progress toward a weight that is smart for you can help diminish or forestall the confusions related with this condition. Your PCP may likewise endorse drugs to deal with certain parts of your concerns related to metabolic conditions. A portion of the ways of diminishing your gamble:

Smart dieting and accomplishing a weight that is good for you assuming that you are overweight or heftiness: Healthy eating and moderate weight reduction, in the scope of 5% to 10% of body weight, can assist with reestablishing your body's capacity to perceive insulin and extraordinarily lessen the opportunity that the condition will turn into a more difficult sickness. This should be possible through diet, exercise, or even with assistance from weight reduction prescriptions whenever suggested by your PCP.
Work out: Increased action alone can further develop your insulin awareness. Oxygen consuming activity, for example, a lively 30-minute everyday walk can advance weight reduction, further developed circulatory strain and fatty substances levels and a diminished gamble of creating diabetes. Most medical care suppliers suggest 150 minutes of oxygen consuming activity every week. Exercise might decrease the gamble for coronary illness even without going with weight reduction. Any expansion in actual work is useful, in any event, for those unfit to perform 150 minutes of action each week.
Dietary changes: Maintain an eating regimen that holds starches to something like half of all our calories. The wellspring of carbs ought to be entire grains (complex carbs, for example, entire grain bread (rather than white) and earthy colored rice (rather than white). Entire grain items alongside vegetables (for instance, beans), leafy foods permit you to have a higher dietary fiber. Eat less red meats and poultry. All things considered, eat more fish (without the skin and not broiled). About a third of your day to day calories ought to come from fat. Consume sound fats, for example, those in canola oil, olive oil, flaxseed oil and tree nuts.

On the off chance that I have a metabolic condition, what medical issues could create?

Reliably elevated degrees of insulin and glucose are connected to numerous unsafe changes to the body, including:

Harm to the covering of coronary and different courses, a critical stage toward the improvement of coronary illness or stroke
Changes in the kidneys' capacity to eliminate salt, prompting hypertension, coronary illness and stroke
An expansion in fatty substance levels, bringing about an expanded gamble of creating cardiovascular illness
An expanded gamble of blood clump development, which can impede corridors and cause coronary failures and strokes
An easing back of insulin creation, which can flag the beginning of type 2 diabetes, a sickness that is in itself related with an expanded gamble for a cardiovascular failure or stroke. Uncontrolled diabetes is likewise connected with entanglements of the eyes, nerves, and kidneys.
Greasy liver, which is some of the time related with irritation of the liver (nonalcoholic steatohepatitis, or NASH). If untreated, NASH could prompt cirrhosis and liver disappointment.

Part four

Effective Treatment for type 2 Diabetes

Chapter nine:

Low- carbohydrate diets

Low-sugar eats less carbs confine
sugar utilization comparative with the typical eating routine. Food varieties high in starches (e.g., sugar, bread, pasta) are restricted, and supplanted with food sources containing a higher level of fat and protein (e.g., meat, poultry, fish, shellfish, eggs, cheddar, nuts, and seeds), as well as low carb food varieties (for example spinach, kale, chard, collards, and other sinewy vegetables).

An illustration of a low-sugar dish, cooked kale and poached eggs
There is an absence of normalization of how much sugar low-starch eats less carbs should have, and this has confounded research.One definition, from the American Academy of Family Physicians, indicates low-carb slims down as having under 20% of calories from carbs.
There is no decent proof that low-starch consuming less calories presents specific medical advantages separated from weight reduction, where low-carb slims down accomplish results like different eating regimens, as weight reduction is not set in stone by calorie limitation and adherence.
An outrageous type of low-starch diet called the ketogenic diet was first settled as a clinical eating regimen for treating epilepsy. It turned into a well known prevailing fashion diet for weight reduction through superstar underwriting, yet there is no proof of any unmistakable advantage for this reason and the eating routine conveys a gamble of unfriendly effects,with the British Dietetic Association naming it one of the "main five most exceedingly terrible celeb diets to stay away from" in 2018.

Macronutrient proportions

The macronutrient proportions of low-sugar eats less are not normalized. Starting around 2018, the clashing meanings of "low-sugar" eats less have muddled examination into the subject. The National Lipid Association and Lifestyle Task force characterize low-starch diets and those containing under 25% of calories from sugars, and exceptionally low carb eats less carbs being those containing under 10% carbohydrates.A 2016 audit of low-carb consumes less calories arranged slims down with 50g of carb each day (under 10% of all out calories) as "extremely low" and diets with 40% of calories from carbs as "gentle" low-carb eats less. The UK National Health Service suggests that "sugars ought to be the body's primary wellspring of energy in a solid, adjusted diet."

Groceries

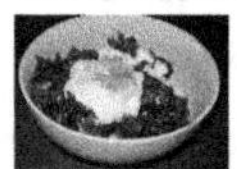

A heap of wavy kale leaves.

Like other verdant vegetables, wavy kale is a food that is low in sugars.

There is proof that the quality, as opposed to the amount, of starch in an eating routine is significant for wellbeing, and that high-fiber slow-processing carb rich food varieties are energizing while exceptionally refined and sweet food sources are less so.People picking diet for ailments ought to have their eating regimen customized to their individual requirements.For individuals with metabolic circumstances, an eating regimen with roughly 40-half carb is suggested.

Most vegetables are low-or moderate-carb food sources (in some low-starch counts calories, fiber is barred in light of the fact that it's anything but a nutritive carb). A few vegetables, like potatoes, carrots, maize (corn) and rice are high in starch. Most low-sugar diet plans oblige vegetables, for example, broccoli, spinach, kale, lettuce, cucumbers, cauliflower, Brussels fledglings, peppers and most green-verdant vegetables.

Chapter Ten

Intermittent fasting

Intermittent fasting, otherwise called discontinuous energy limitation, is any of different dinner timing plans that cycle between intentional fasting (or decreased calorie consumption) and non-fasting over a given period. Techniques for irregular fasting incorporate substitute day fasting,periodic fasting, and day to day time-confined taking care of.

Discontinuous fasting might have comparative impacts to a calorie-limitation diet,and has been concentrated on as of late as a training to perhaps decrease the gamble of diet-related illnesses, for example, metabolic syndrome.The American Heart Association expresses that irregular fasting might create weight reduction, diminish insulin obstruction, and lower the gamble of cardiometabolic infections, despite the fact that its drawn out supportability is obscure. A 2019 survey reasoned that irregular fasting might assist with corpulence, insulin obstruction, dyslipidemia, hypertension, and irritation. A 2022 survey showed that irregular fasting is by and large safe.Adverse impacts of discontinuous fasting have not been thoroughly considered, driving a few scholastics to bring up its gamble as a dietary fad.The US National Institute on Aging states that there is lacking proof to suggest discontinuous fasting, and urges addressing one's medical services supplier about the advantages and dangers prior to rolling out any critical improvements to one's eating design.

Fasting exists in different strict works on, including Buddhism, Christianity, Hinduism, Islam, Jainism and Judaism.

Kinds of discontinuous fasting

Three techniques for discontinuous fasting are time-confined taking care of, substitute day fasting, and occasional fasting:

1. Time-confined taking care includes eating just during a specific number of hours every day, frequently laying out a reliable day to day example of caloric admission inside a

8-12-hour time window. This timetable might adjust food admission to circadian rhythms.

2. Substitute day fasting includes shifting back and forth between a 24-hour "quick day" when the individual eats under 25% of normal energy needs, trailed by a 24-hour non-fasting "feast day" time frame. It is the strictest type of irregular fasting since there are more long stretches of fasting per week.There are two subtypes:
    - Complete substitute day fasting (or all out discontinuous energy limitation), where no calories are consumed on fasting days.
    - Changed substitute day fasting (or fractional discontinuous energy limitation) which permits the utilization of up to 25% of everyday calorie needs on fasting days rather than complete fasting. This is similar to exchanging days with ordinary eating and days with an exceptionally low-calorie diet.

Intermittent fasting or entire day fasting includes any time of back to back fasting of over 24 hours, for example, the 5:2 eating regimen where there are a couple of fasting days of the week, to the more outrageous rendition with a few days or long stretches of fasting.During the fasting days, utilization of roughly 500 to 700 calories, or around 25% of normal day to day caloric admission, might be permitted rather than complete fasting.

The science concerning discontinuous fasting is primer and dubious because of a shortfall of concentrates on its drawn out effects.Preliminary proof shows that irregular fasting might be successful for weight reduction, may diminish insulin obstruction and fasting insulin, and may work on cardiovascular and metabolic wellbeing, albeit the drawn out supportability of these impacts has not been considered.

www.ingramcontent.com/pod-product-compliance
Lightning Source LLC
LaVergne TN
LVHW052102160826
845678LV00015B/3323

* 9 7 9 8 3 5 1 2 3 4 8 3 0 *